SQUASH BOOM BEET

an alphabet for healthy, adventurous eaters

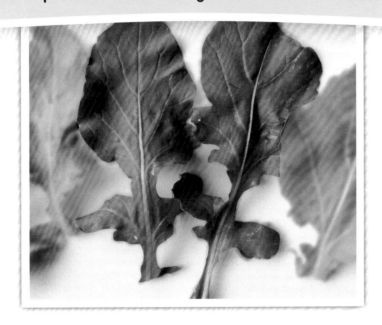

To Debbie,
Thanks for raising
a healthy daughter!
Lisa M. Price

BLUE
BAY
BOOKS

Squash Boom Beet: An Alphabet For Healthy, Adventurous Eaters
Written and Photographed by Lisa Maxbauer Price

Design by Bethany Gulde, Bethany Design, www.bethanydesigntc.com
Copy Editing by Tara Hans
Special Consultants: Michael Lancashire (photography), Bob Smith (Book Printers Network) and David Hilt (technology)
Printing and Binding by Bang Printing, Brainerd, MN, www.bangprinting.com

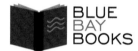

BLUE BAY BOOKS

Published by Blue Bay Books
Traverse City, Michigan

All inquiries should be addressed to:
Blue Bay Books
P.O. Box 214
Traverse City, MI 49685
Email: info@bluebaybooks.com

For book ordering information or to purchase photographs from the book, visit:
www.bluebaybooks.com
www.squashboombeet.com

Special thanks to…
Grand Traverse Area Catholic Schools, where I learned to read;
Saint Mary's College, where I began to write;
First for Women magazine, where I put it all together. -LMP

First Edition

Made in the U.S.A.

Proudly made in Michigan and printed in the Midwest
at Bang Printing, an environmentally responsible
Green Initiative Certified press. Printed using soy oil inks.

Printed ISBN: 978-0-9968530-0-2

Library of Congress Control Number: 2015918465

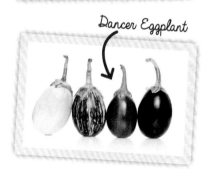

Peaches and Cream Corn

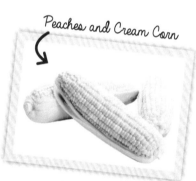

Ginger

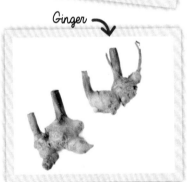

Dancer Eggplant

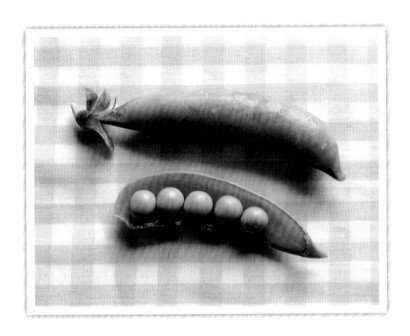

To my three little peas:

Jackson P, Dashiell P & Xavier P

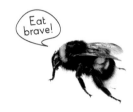

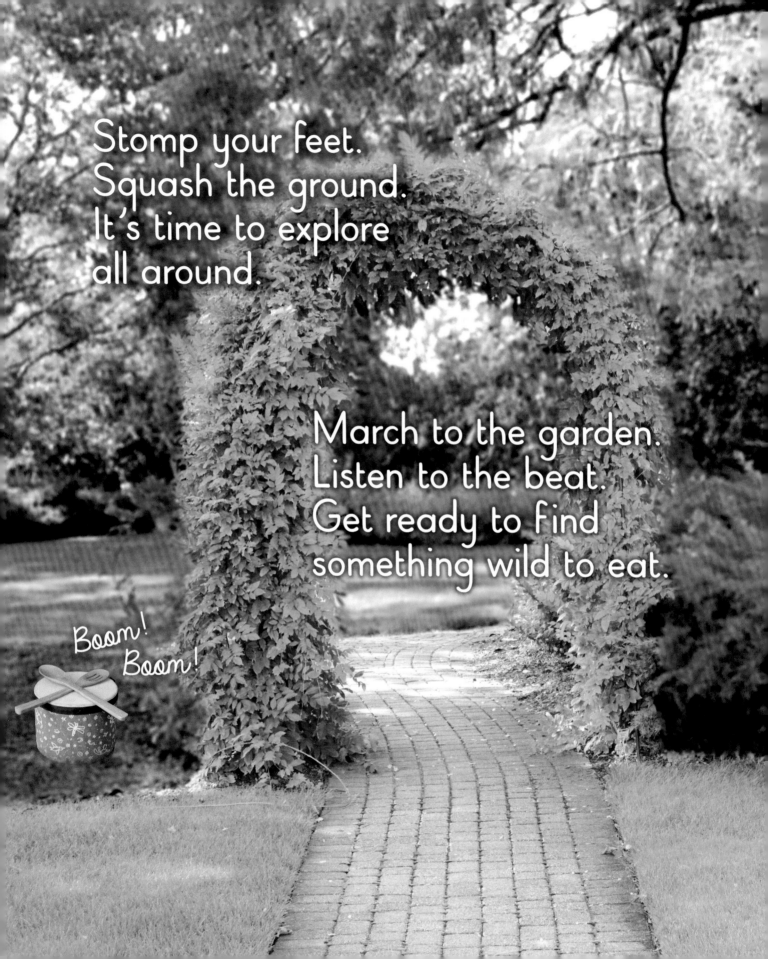

Stomp your feet.
Squash the ground.
It's time to explore
all around.

March to the garden.
Listen to the beat.
Get ready to find
something wild to eat.

Boom!
Boom!

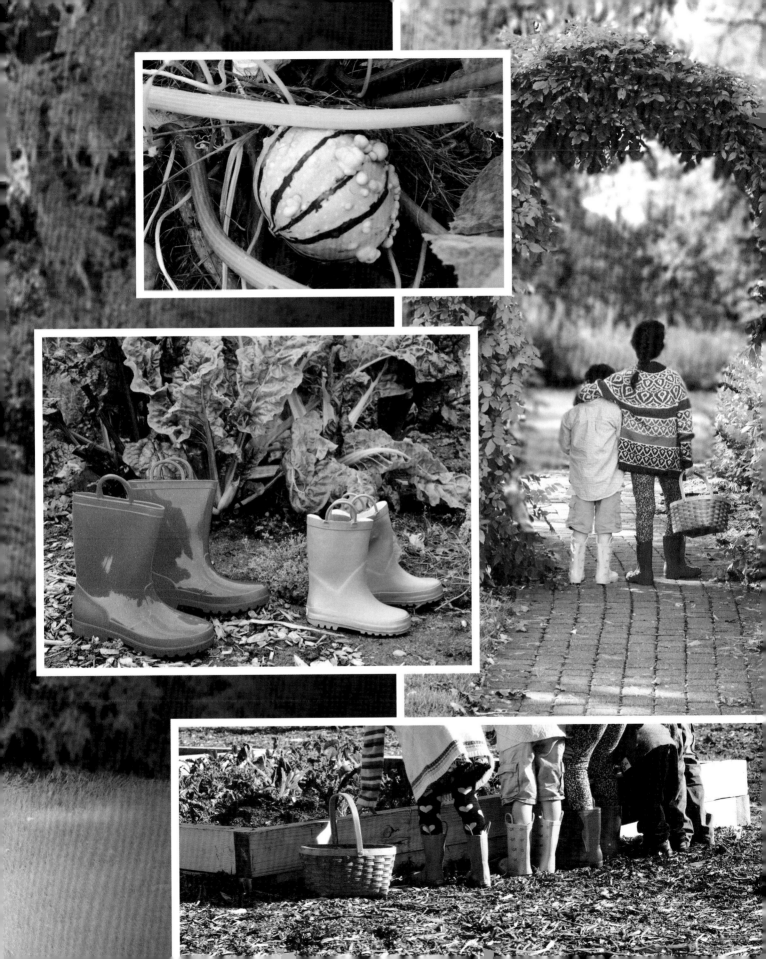

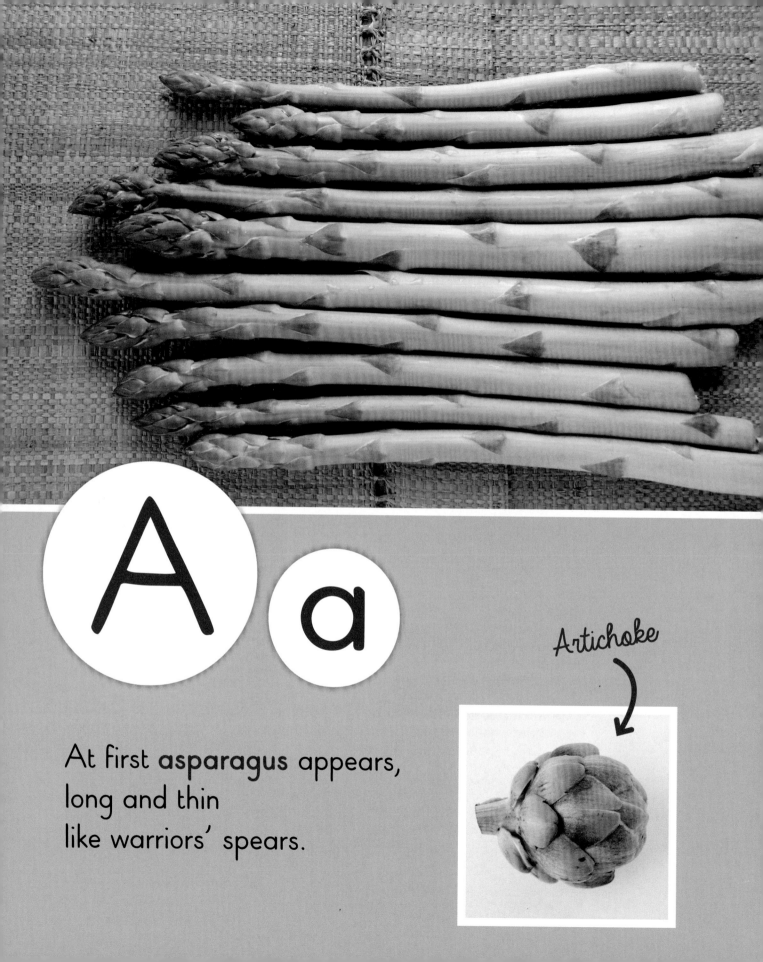

A a

Artichoke

At first **asparagus** appears,
long and thin
like warriors' spears.

Candy Cane Beets

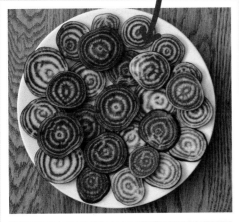

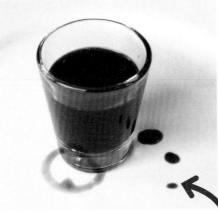

Beet Juice

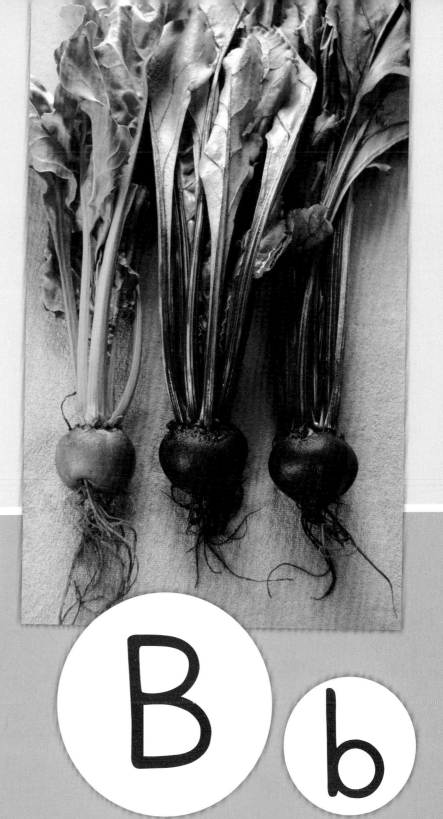

B b

Then marvelous **beets**, with juice like ink.
Better wash after eating in the nearest sink.

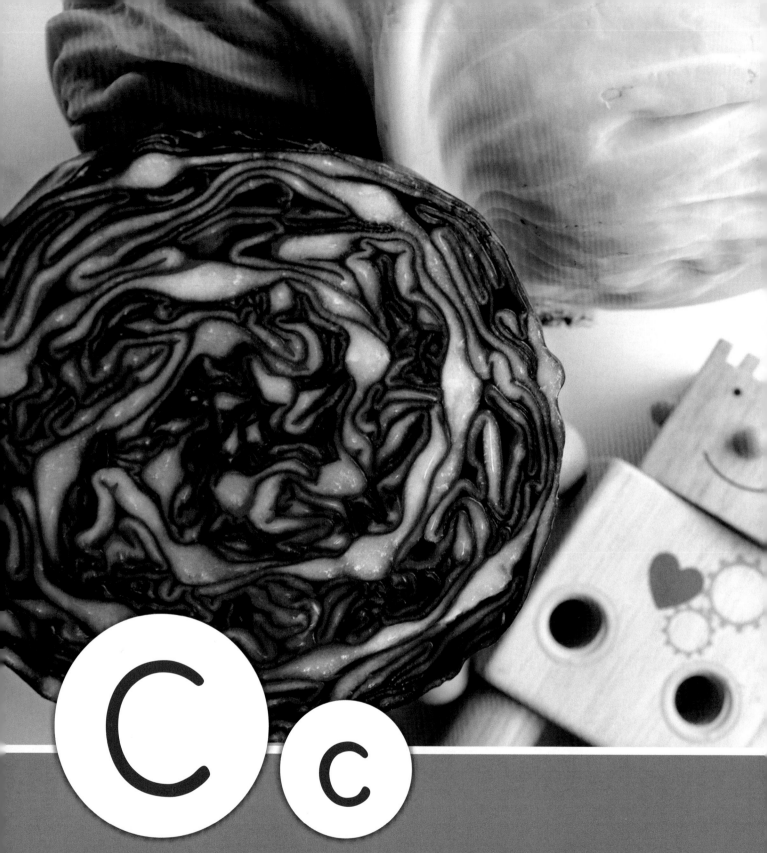

Cc

Slice through cabbage and it looks like brain.
Robots don't have one, so they can't explain.

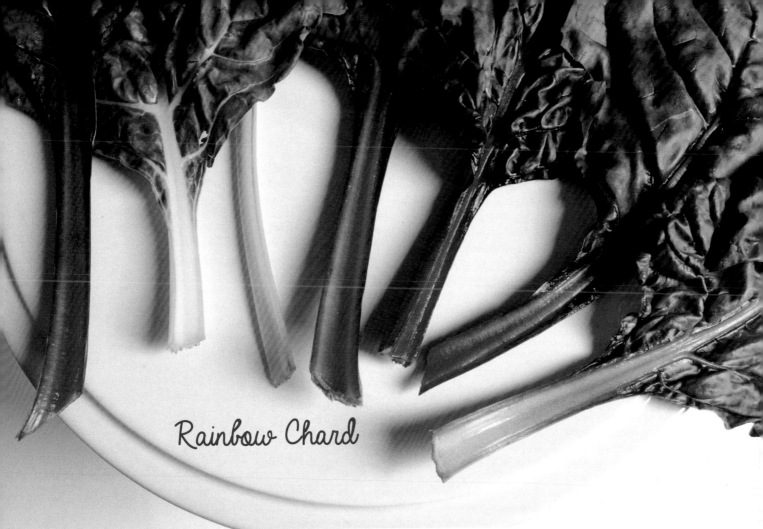

Rainbow Chard

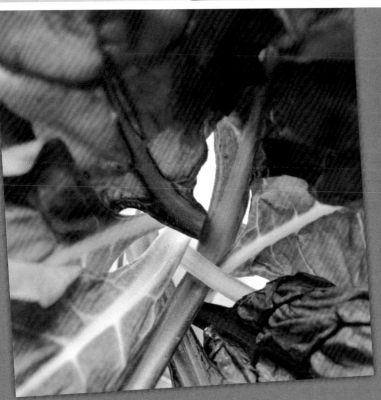

You will know
Swiss chard by its
rainbow stems
that are found on its
wildly colorful ends.

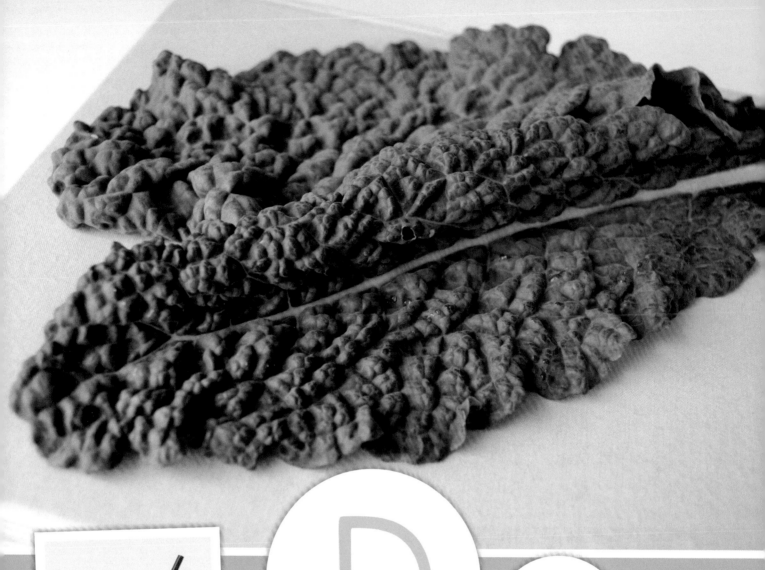

D d

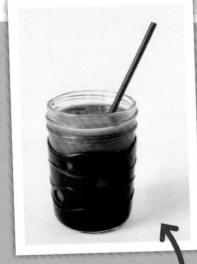

Green Drink

Dinosaur kale feels like an elephant's wrinkled skin. Watch leaves turn to liquid after a blender spin.

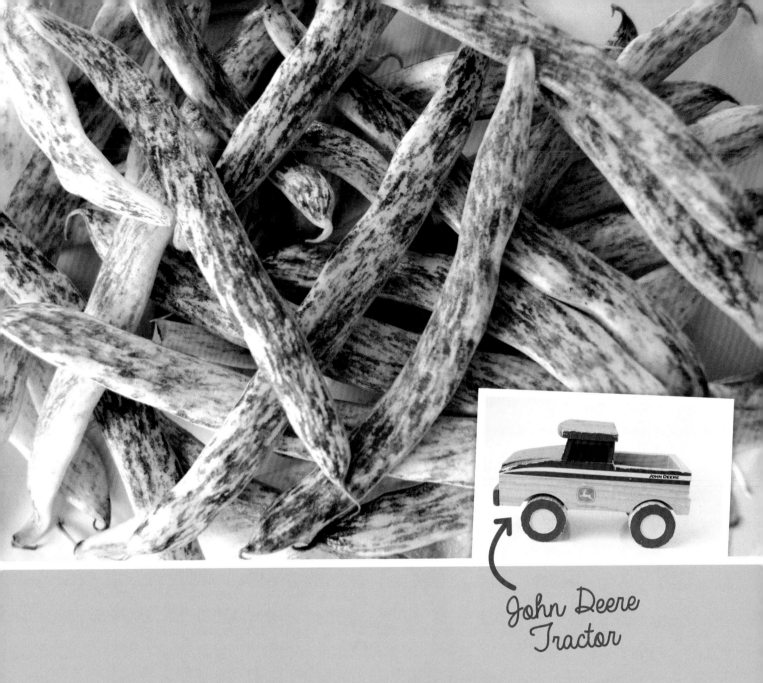

John Deere
Tractor

See the dragon tongue beans?
No need to fear!
Cook them to make those
odd purple spots disappear.

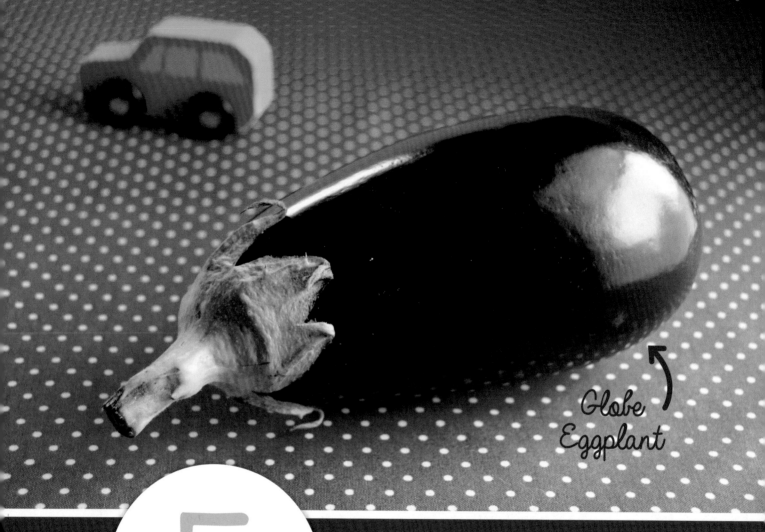

Globe Eggplant

E e

Don't let eggplant's spiny stems deter.
Its fleshy fruit has a nice meaty texture.

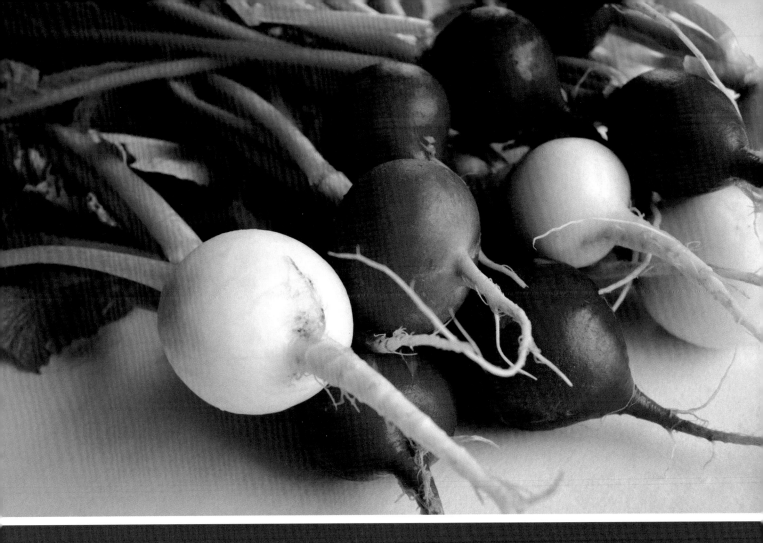

Easter egg radishes are known far and wide for looking this festive without being dyed.

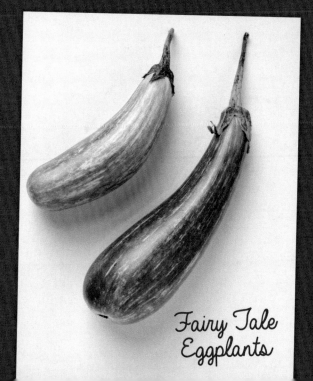

Fairy Tale Eggplants

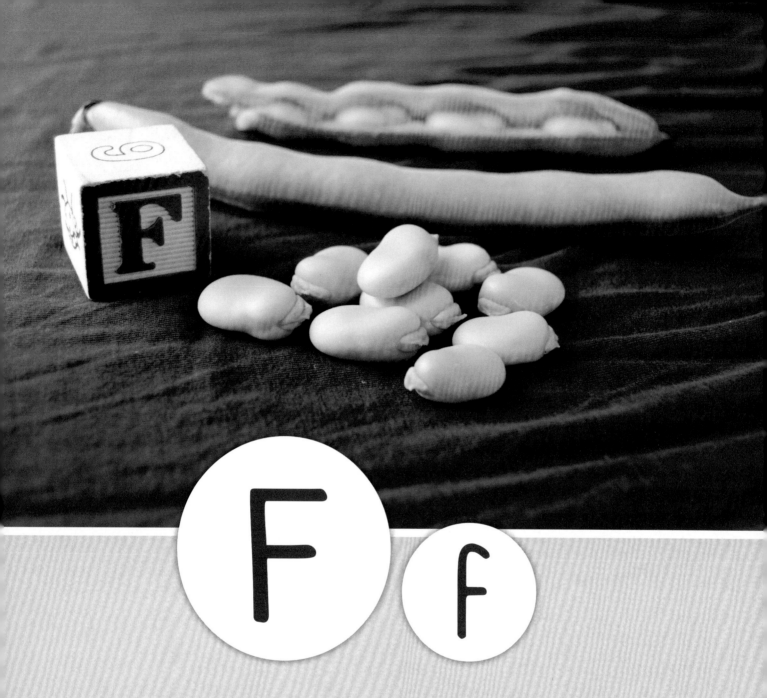

Tucked inside **fava bean's** pillowy pod bed
is a second shell to shed before you can be fed.

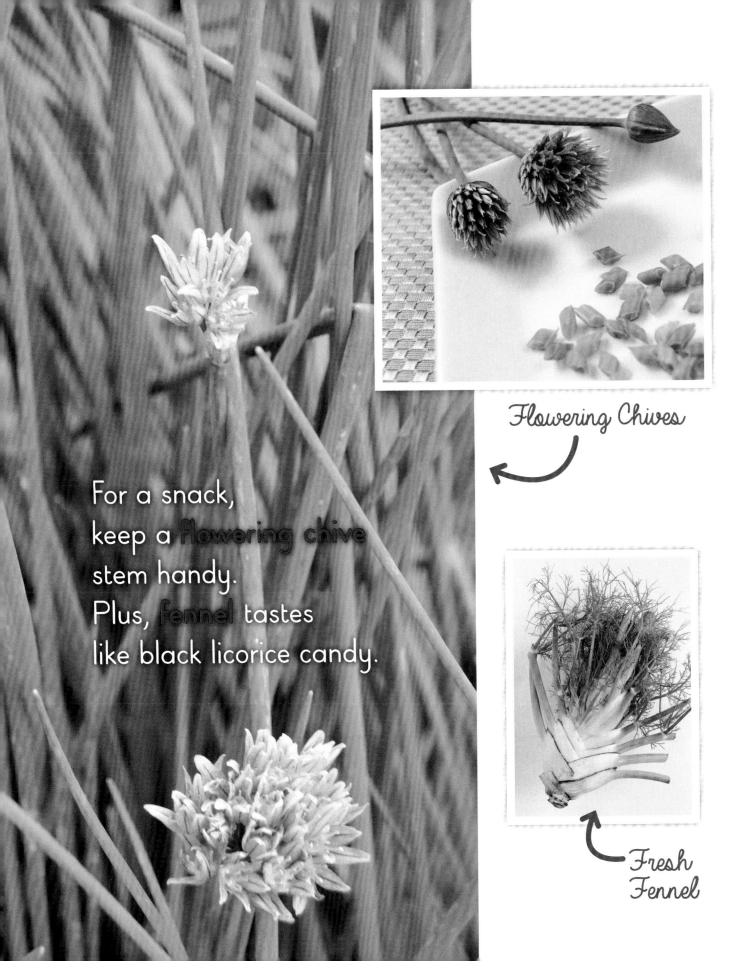

For a snack,
keep a flowering chive
stem handy.
Plus, fennel tastes
like black licorice candy.

Flowering Chives

Fresh
Fennel

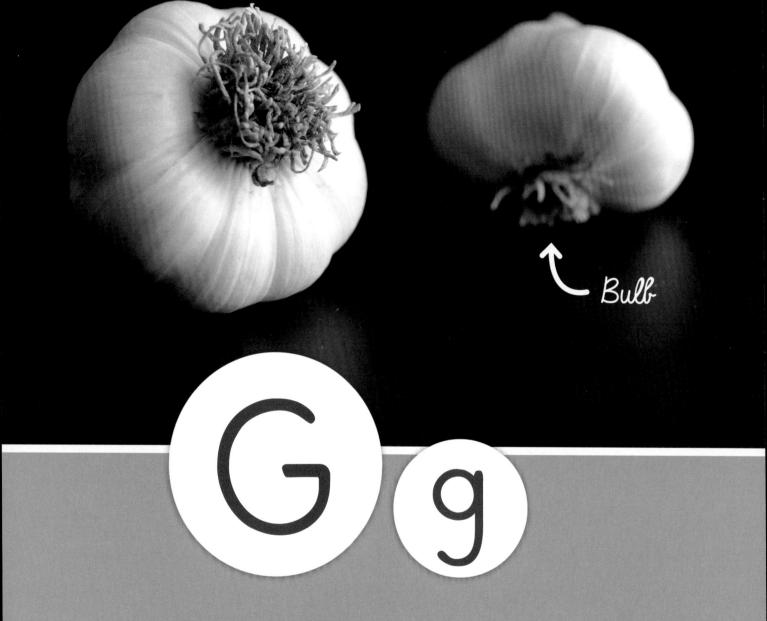

Bulb

G g

Garlic may be stinky, but eat it every day.
It might keep the doctor (or Dracula) away.

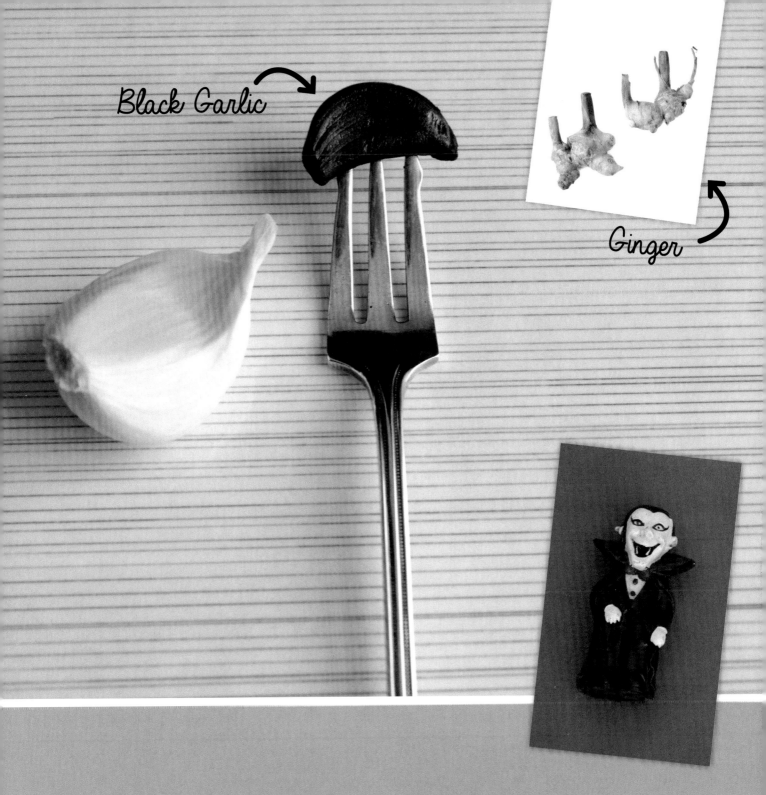

Black Garlic

Ginger

Peel to study a bulb's papery skin
or chew a black clove like a vitamin.

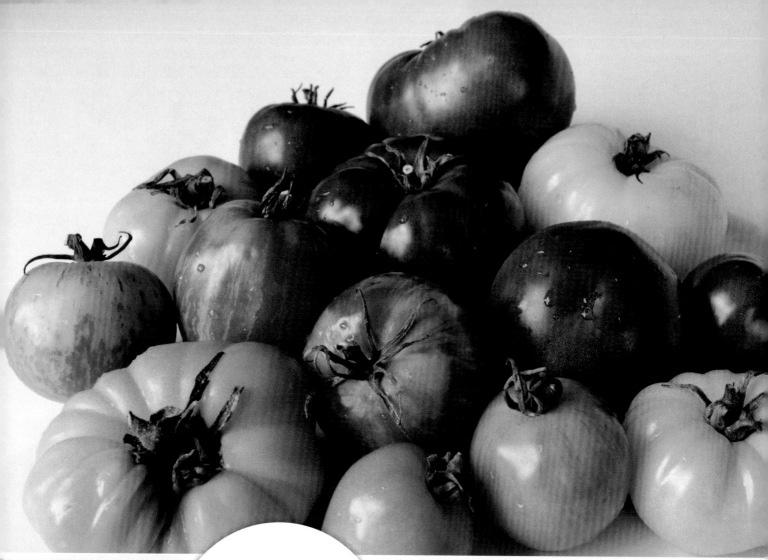

H h

Heaps of heirloom tomatoes, knobby and strange,
grow not just in red, their hue can change.

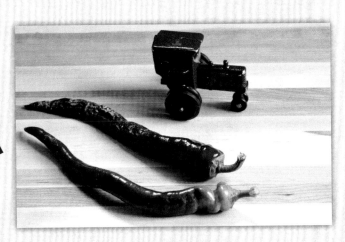

Hot Peppers

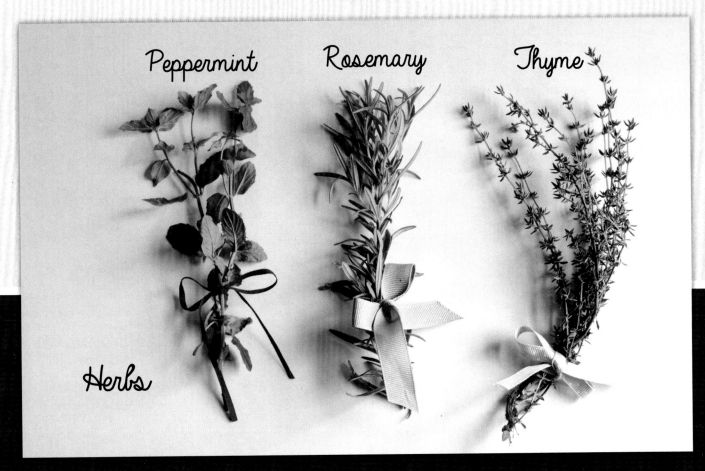

Peppermint   Rosemary   Thyme

Herbs

You can also eat thyme, no not from a clock.
The **healing herb** is used in sauce and soup stock.

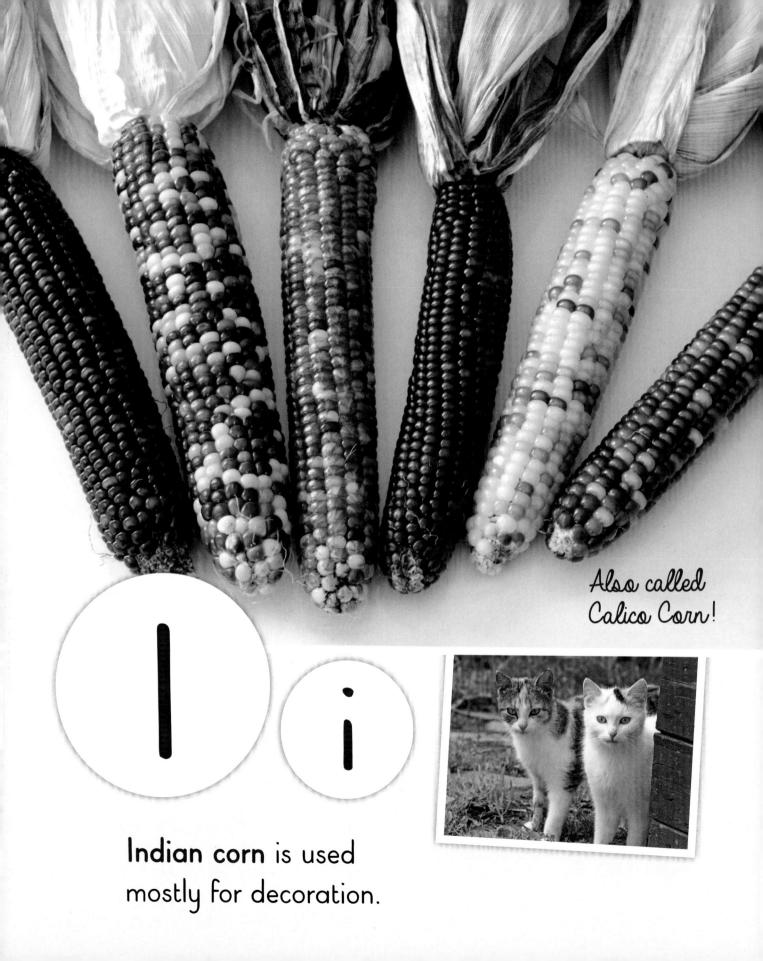

*Also called
Calico Corn!*

I i

Indian corn is used
mostly for decoration.

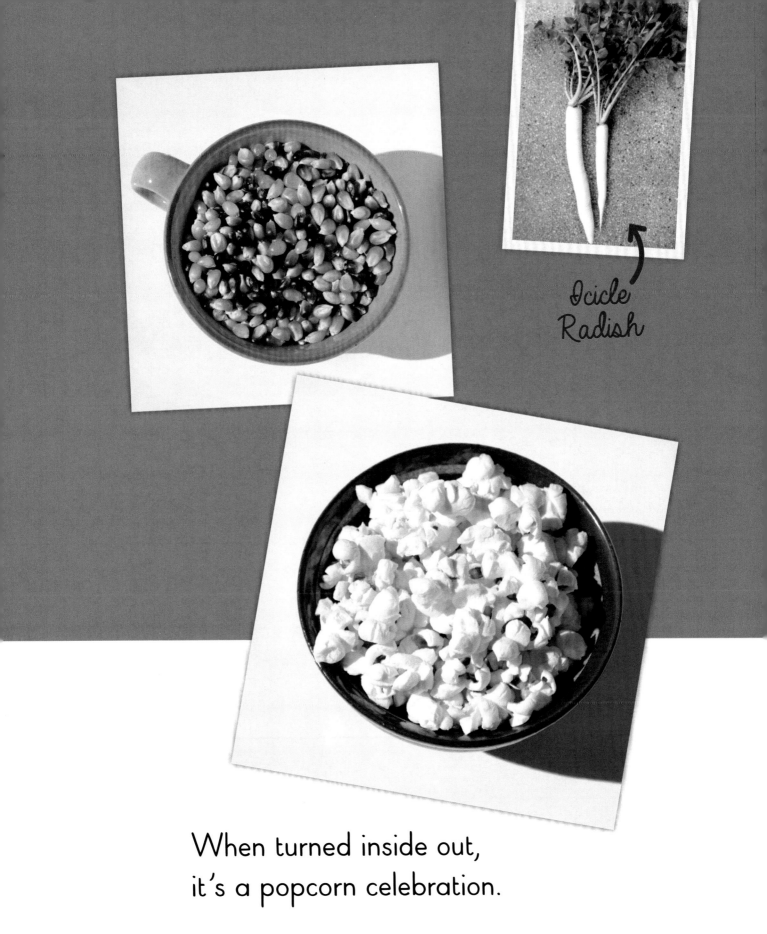

Icicle
Radish

When turned inside out,
it's a popcorn celebration.

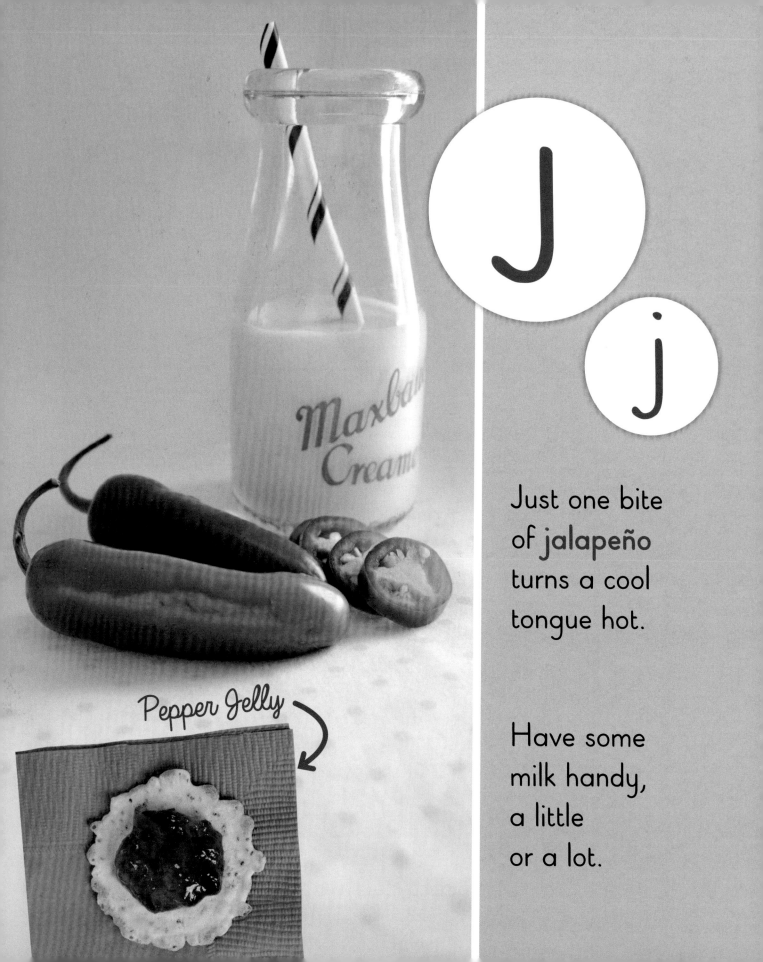

J j

Just one bite
of **jalapeño**
turns a cool
tongue hot.

Have some
milk handy,
a little
or a lot.

Pepper Jelly

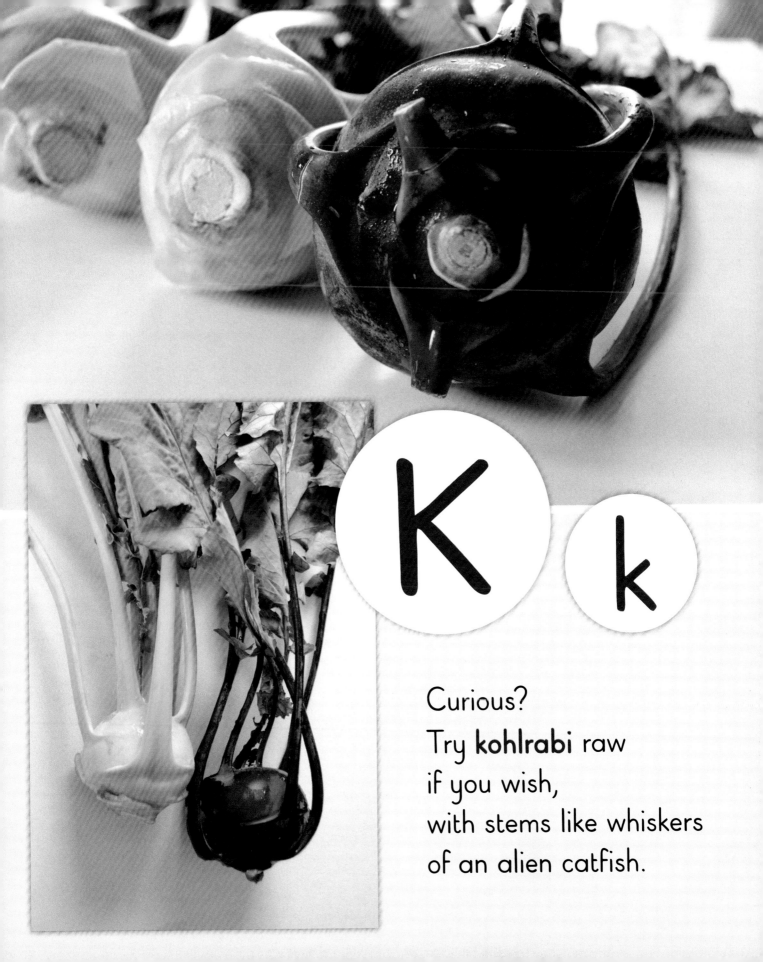

K k

Curious?
Try **kohlrabi** raw
if you wish,
with stems like whiskers
of an alien catfish.

Red Fire Lettuce

Lemon Squash

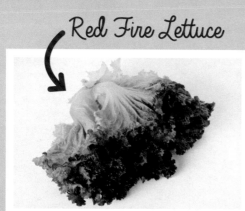

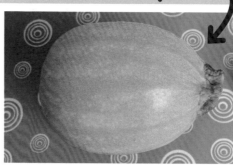

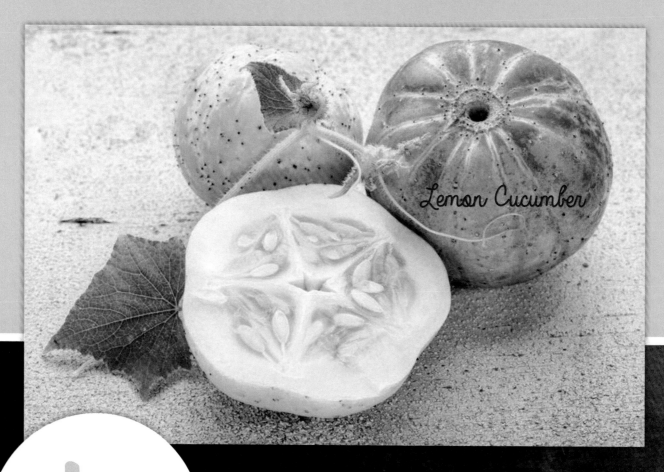

Lemon Cucumber

L l

It won't make you pucker.
The name is a fluke.
But please slice and savor
this round **lemon cuke.**

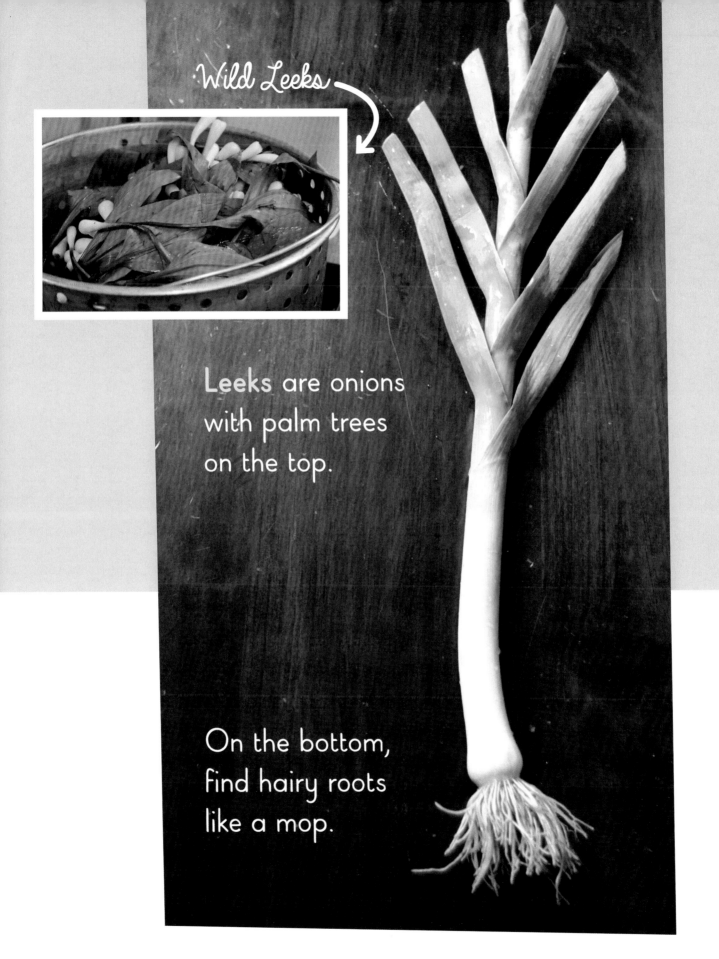

Wild Leeks

Leeks are onions with palm trees on the top.

On the bottom, find hairy roots like a mop.

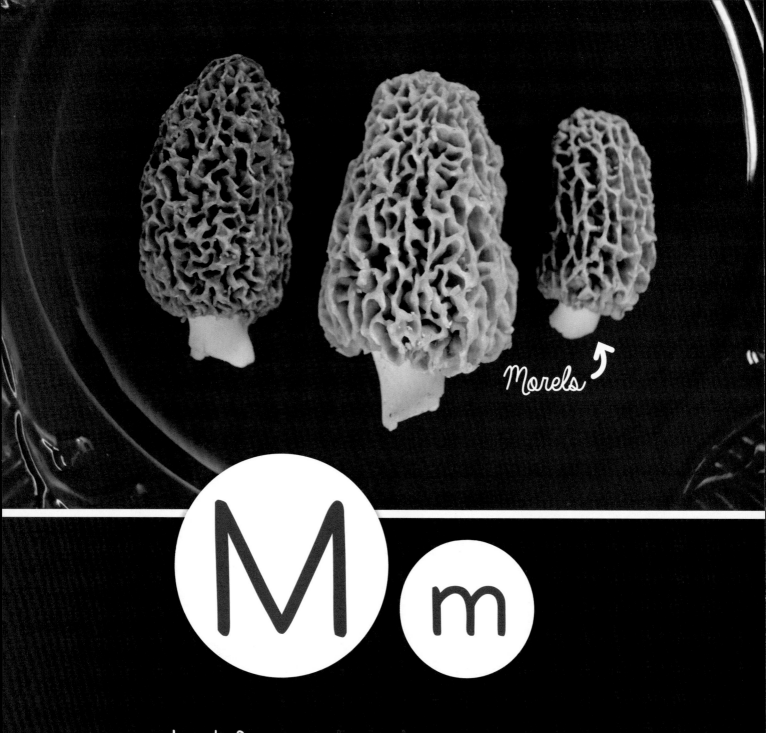

Morels

M m

Look for morel mushrooms
hiding on the forest floor.

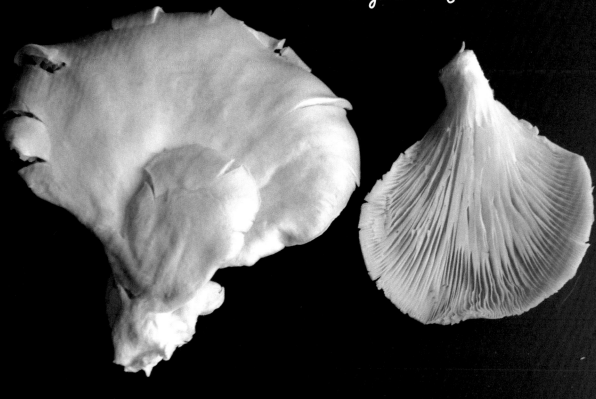

Oyster Mushrooms

Market Basket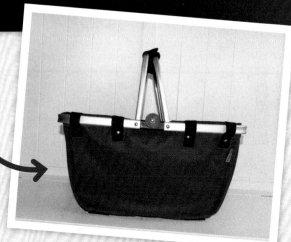

Nn

Nasturtium offers more than gentle perfume.
On salad you can eat this peppery bloom.

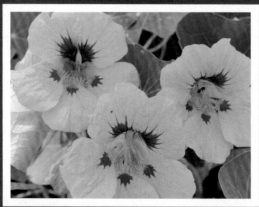 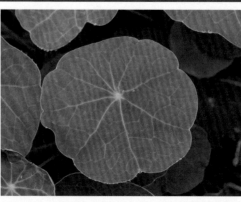

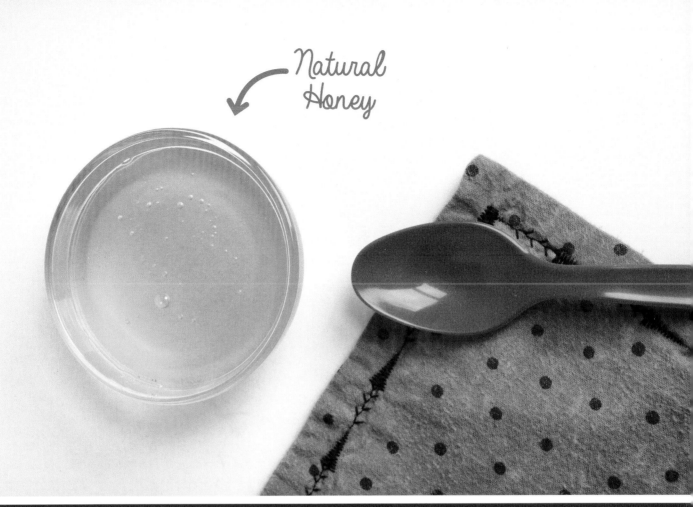

Natural Honey

News flash!
Sweet natural honey will never go rotten.
Thank hardworking bees.
They should not be forgotten.

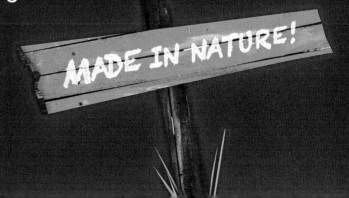

MADE IN NATURE!

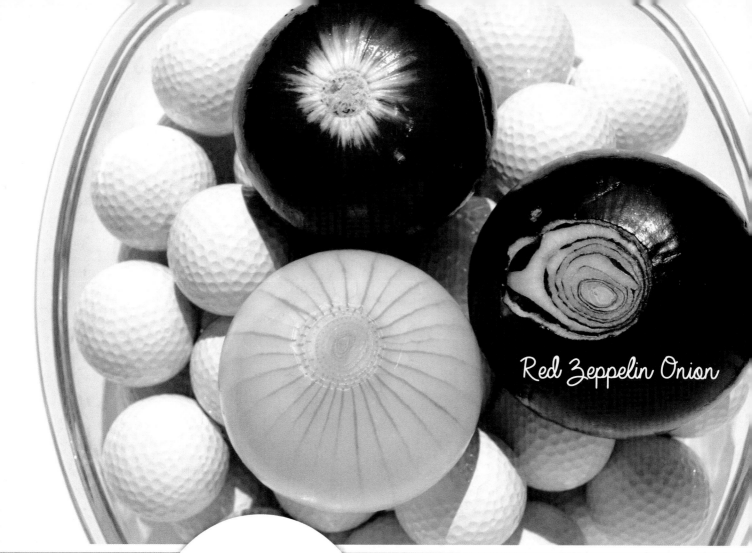

Red Zeppelin Onion

O o

On your mark, get set,
count **onion** layers in one try.
Careful! These vegetables
can make even strong chefs cry.

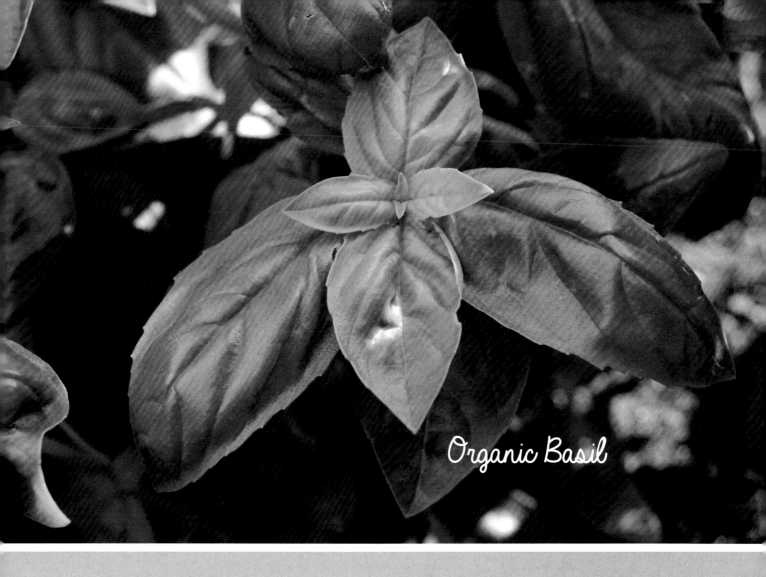

Organic Basil

Organic means food is chemical-free,
just the way nature meant it to be.

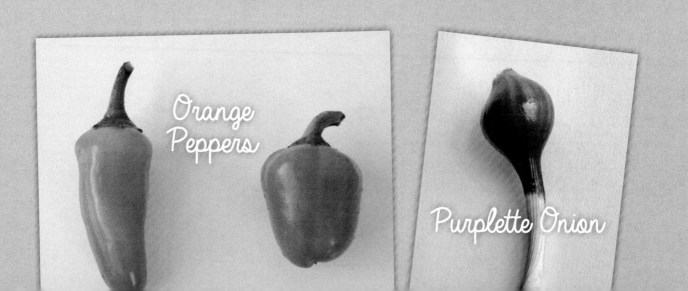

Orange
Peppers

Purplette Onion

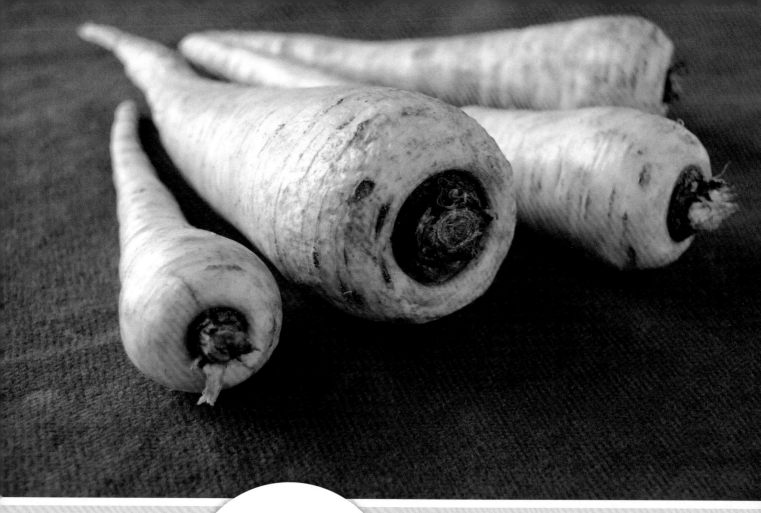

P p

The longer a **parsnip** grows underground,
the sweeter it will be when it's time to chow down.

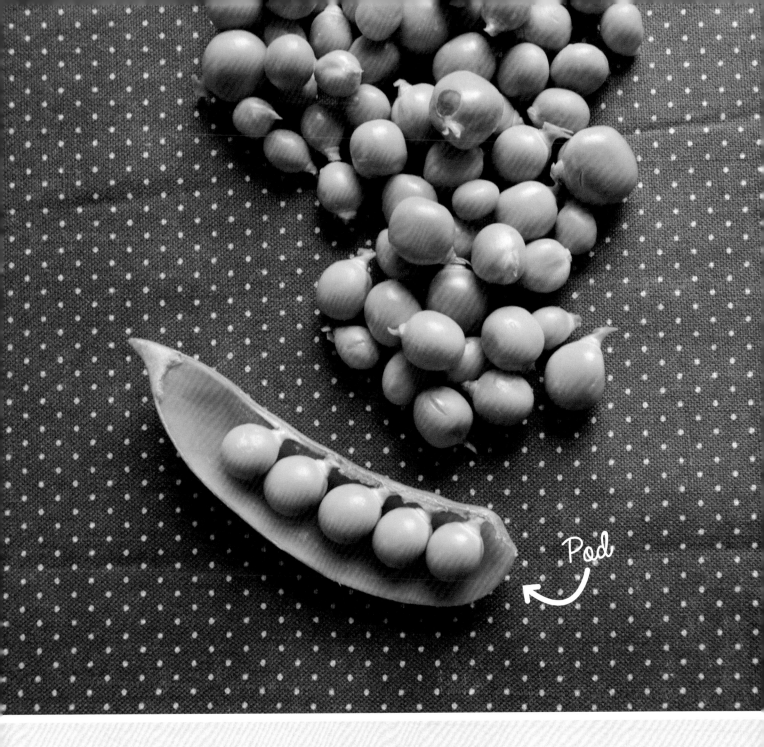

Pod

Boom-boom yippee!
Behold the small but mighty **pea**.
Don't stop now.
Keep reading, look and see...

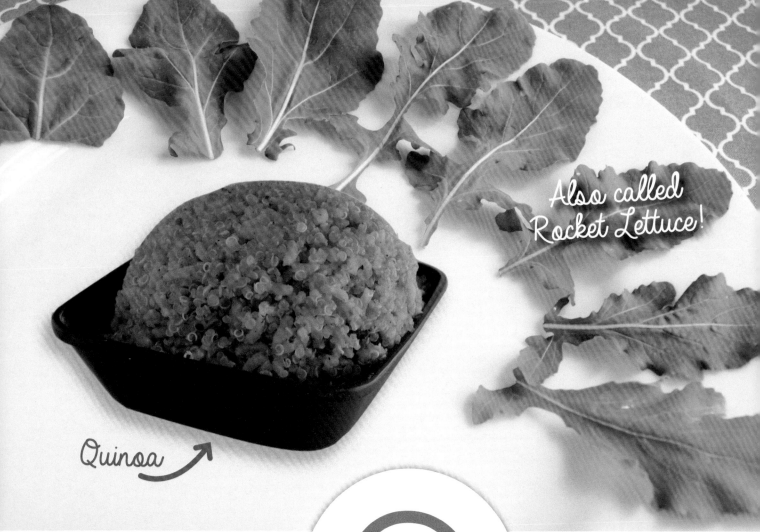

Also called
Rocket Lettuce!

Quinoa →

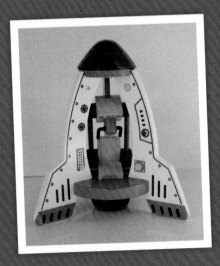

Q q

Protein-powered quinoa
is a very old grain.
So many ways to eat it,
it is totally insane!

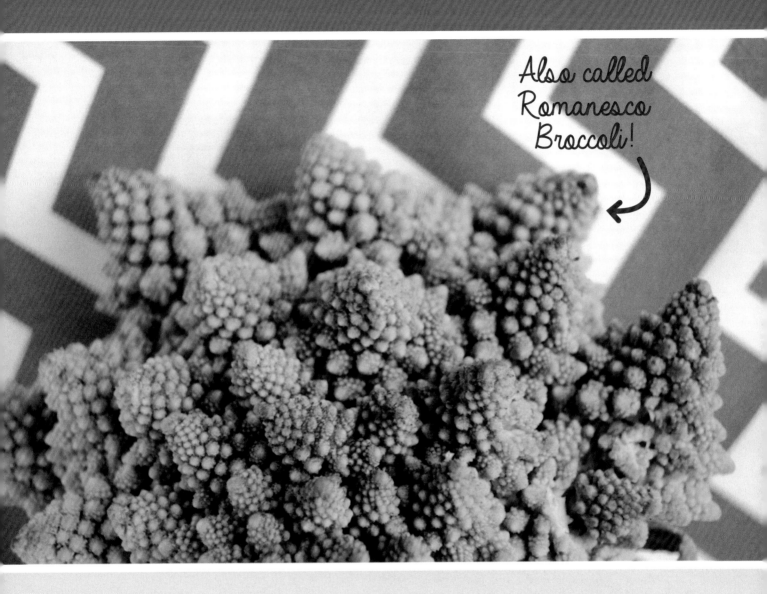

Also called Romanesco Broccoli!

Roquette arugula leaves
grow quite quickly from the ground.
And romanesque cauliflower
looks like a funky queen's crown.

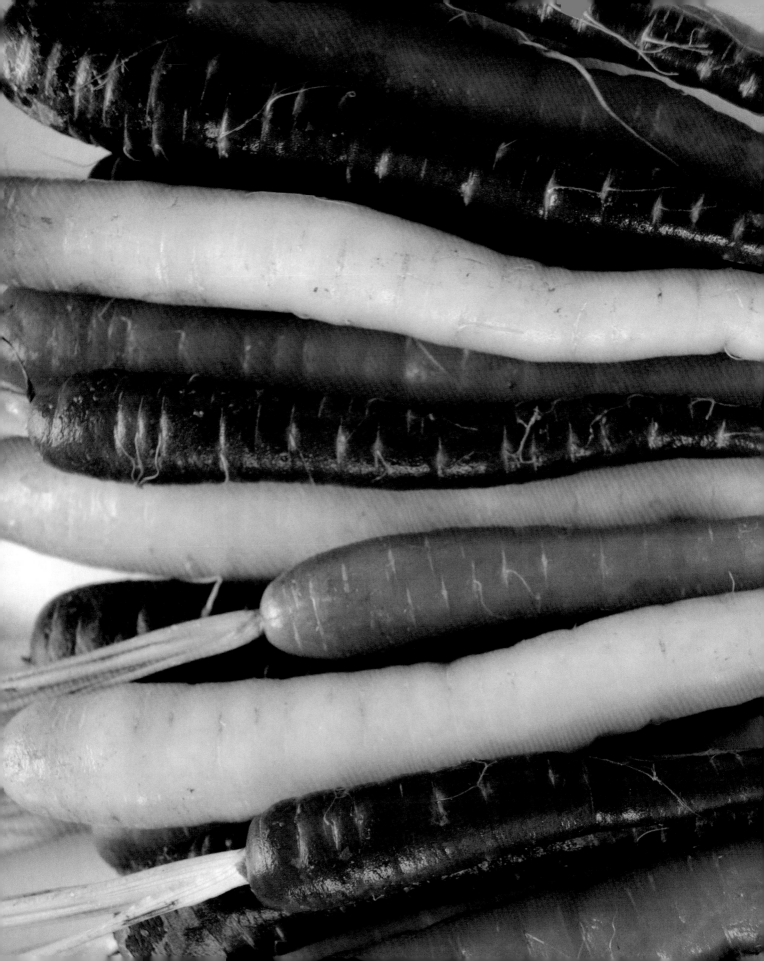

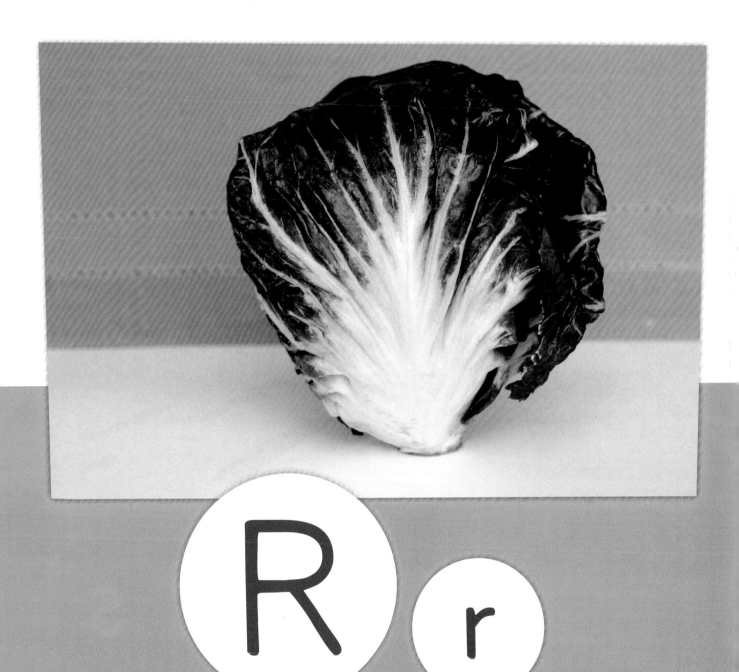

R r

Chilled or grilled, rainbow carrots are unique.
And radicchio has veins like a lightning streak.

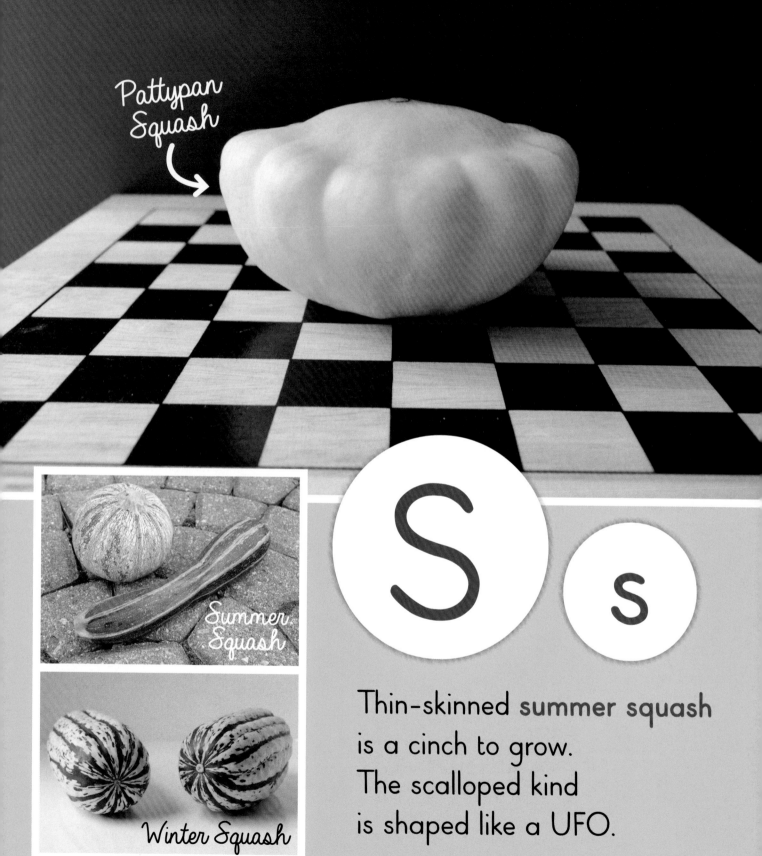

Pattypan
Squash

Summer
Squash

Winter Squash

S s

Thin-skinned **summer squash**
is a cinch to grow.
The scalloped kind
is shaped like a UFO.

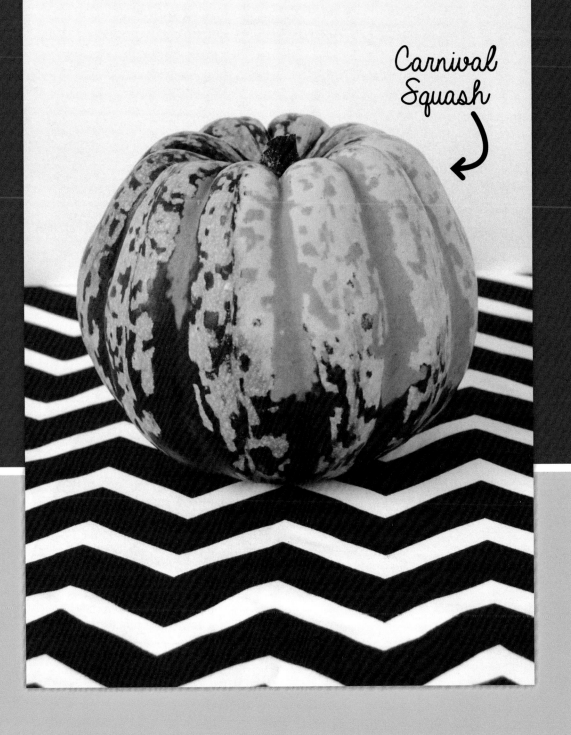

Carnival
Squash

Cooked **winter squash** gives the heart a flutter
when a fork can poke the rind as easily as butter.

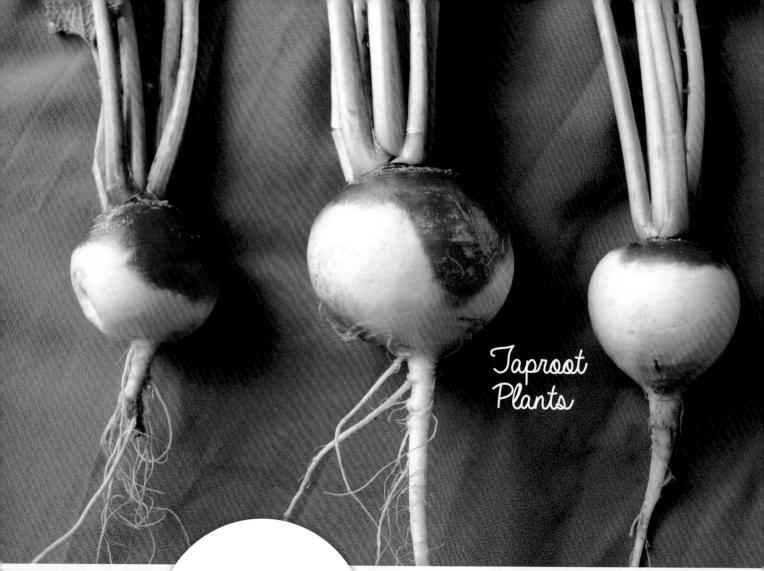

Taproot Plants

T t

A **turnip** is white under dirt where it lays.
The top changes color when touched by sun's rays.

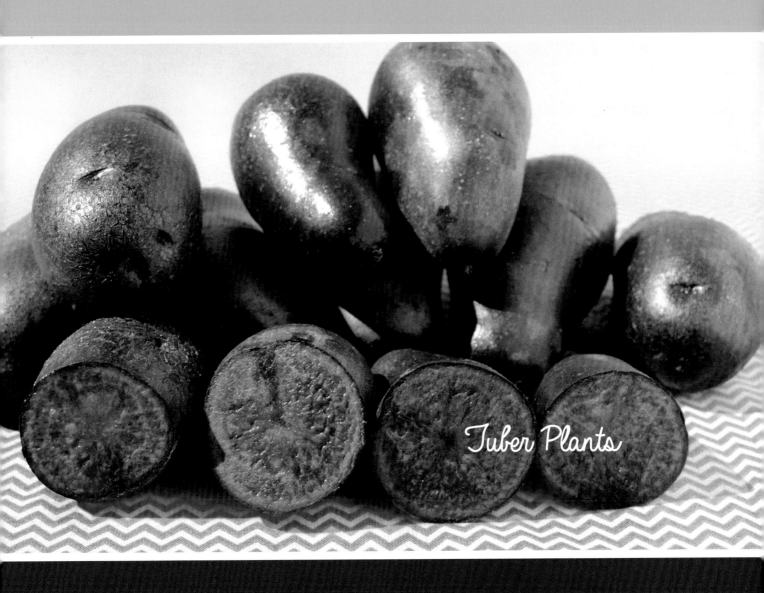

Tuber Plants

It's wise to eat these
purple tater plants.
The fingerlings have tons
of antioxidants.

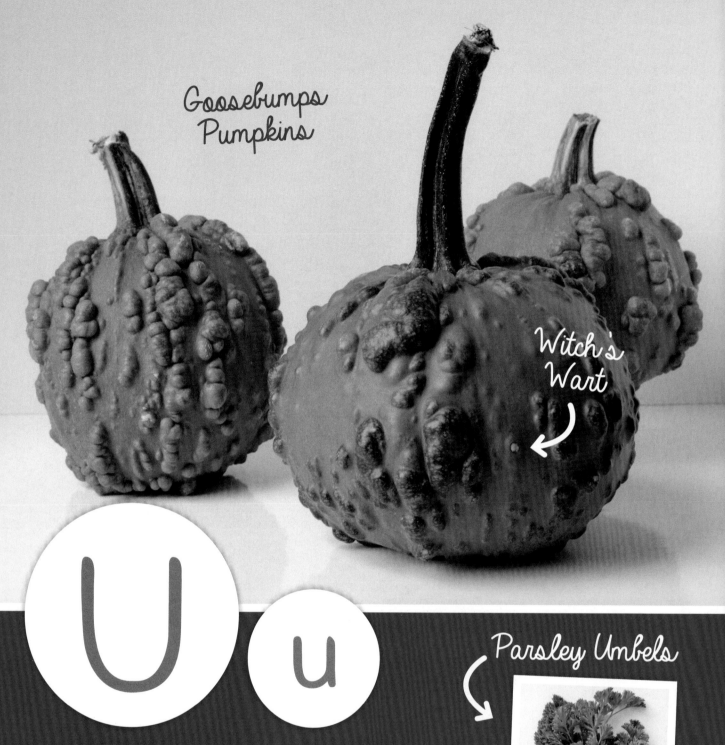

Goosebumps
Pumpkins

Witch's
Wart

U u

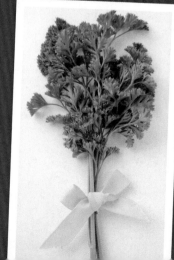

Parsley Umbels

Ugly pumpkins seem scary,
but they are helpful at lunch.
Simply bake the gourd's seeds
for something yummy to crunch.

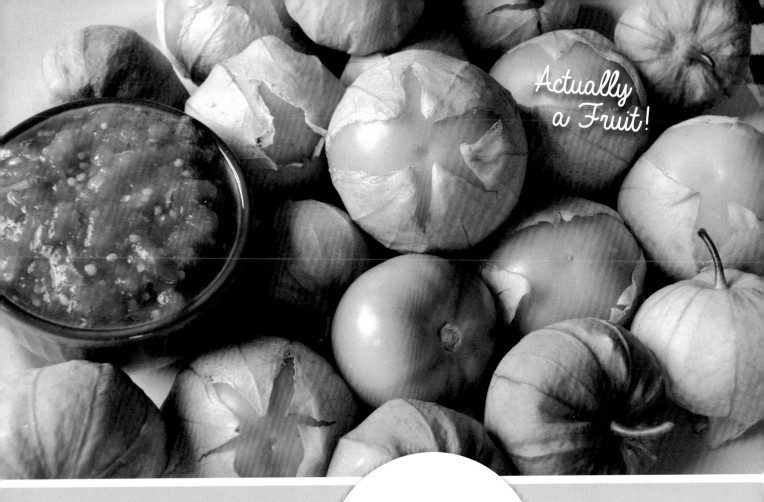

Actually
a Fruit!

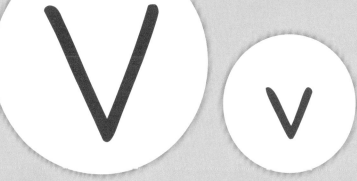

Vine-Ripened
Tomatoes

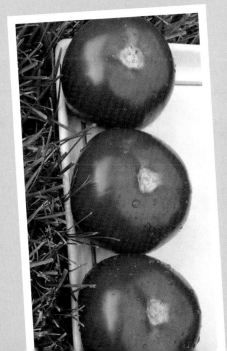

V v

Spy the star on this veggie.
Chip chip hooray!
Tomatillos make very tasty
salsa verde.

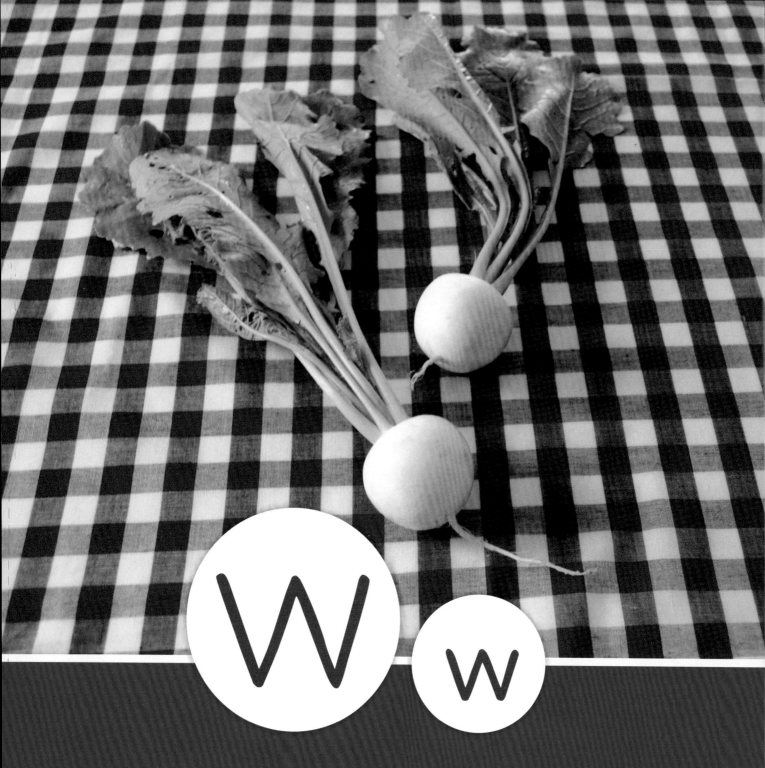

Ww

Wow, the leaves from white salad turnips are sour, but these greens are packed with bone-building power.

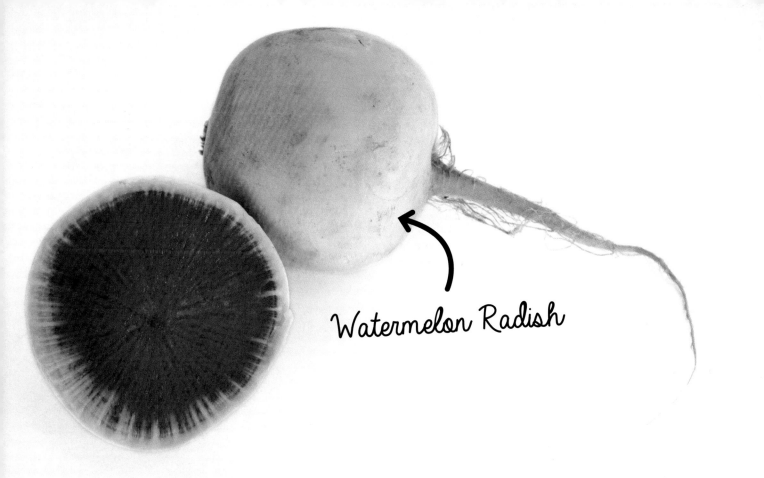

Watermelon Radish

Waste Compost Bin

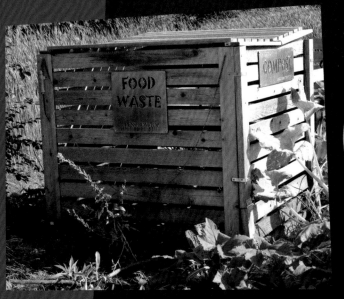

White Squash

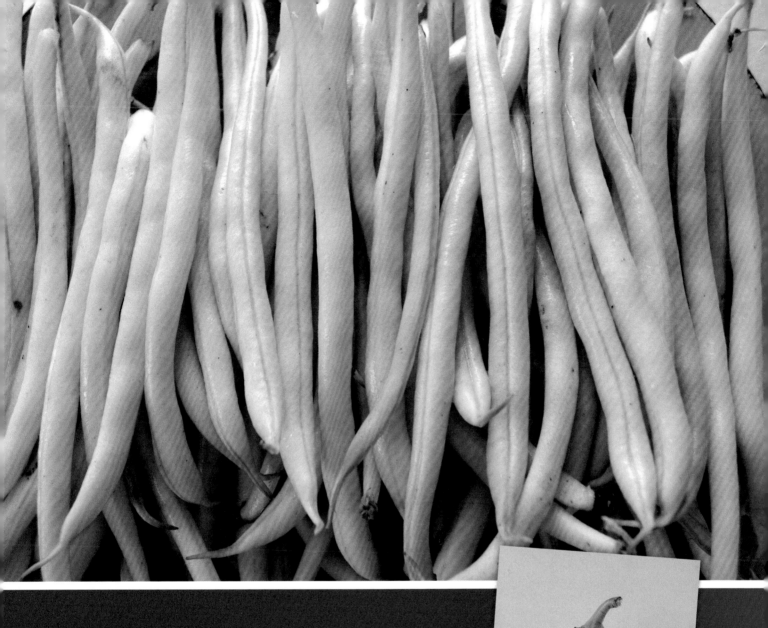

Mixed greens
and wax beans,
there's no question,
they protect tummies
by helping with digestion.

Hot Wax
Pepper

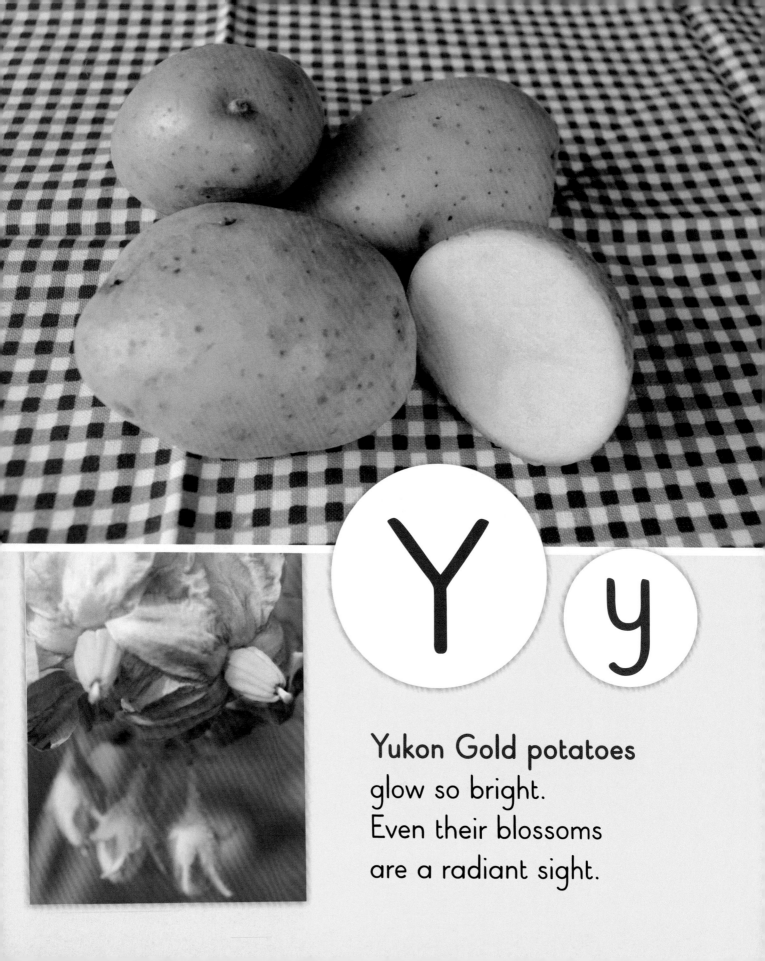

Y y

Yukon Gold potatoes
glow so bright.
Even their blossoms
are a radiant sight.

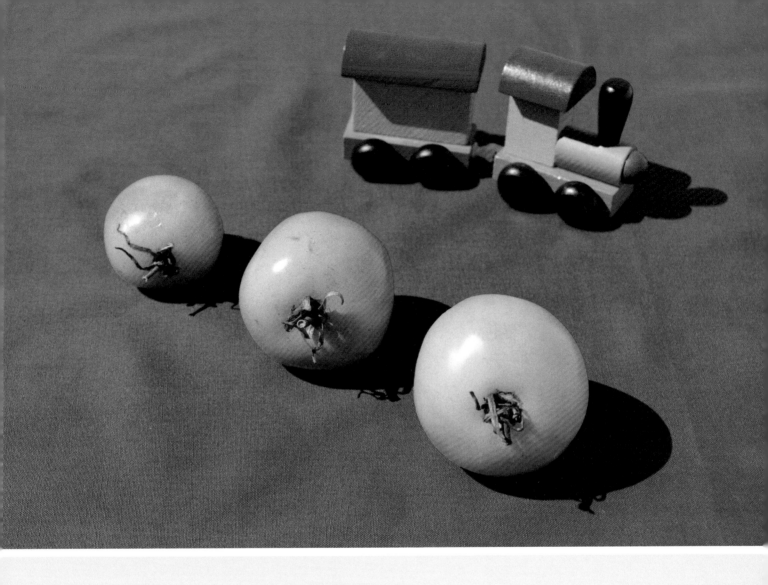

Once a **yellow tomato** begins to sprout,
its climbing vine grows up, not out.

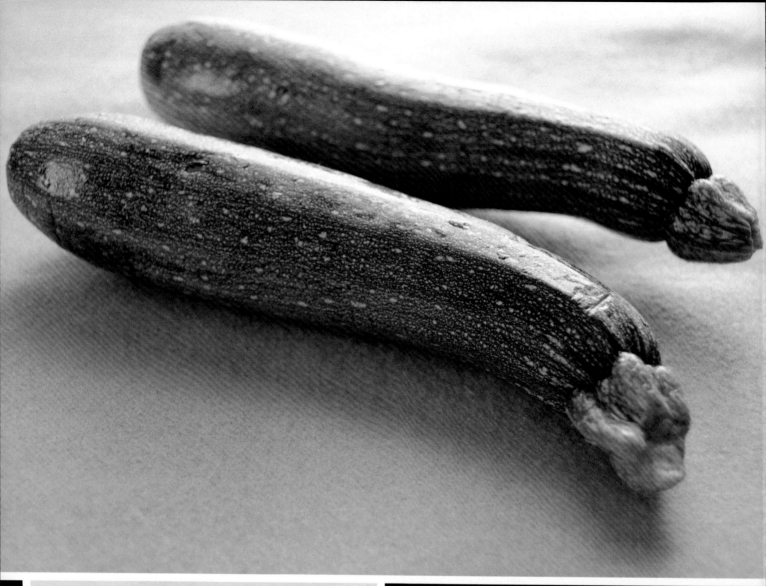

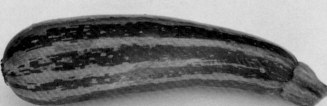

Green Tiger Zucchini

Z z

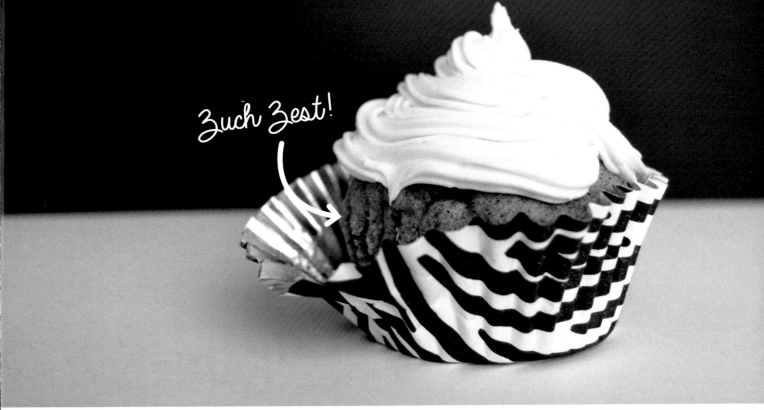

Zuch Zest!

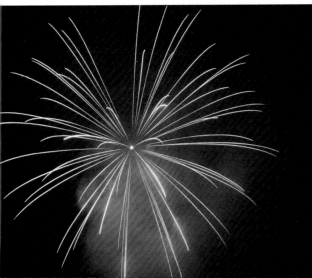

Saved the best for last.
Alert! Alert!
Zucchini is a farm food
you can eat for dessert!

So remember...

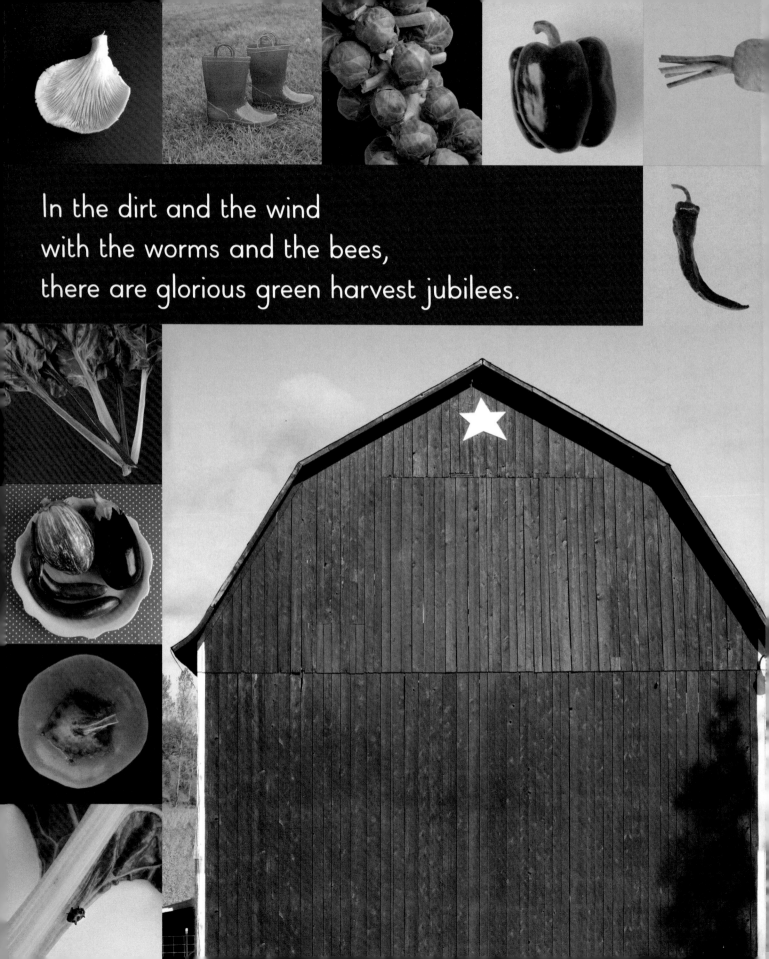

In the dirt and the wind
with the worms and the bees,
there are glorious green harvest jubilees.

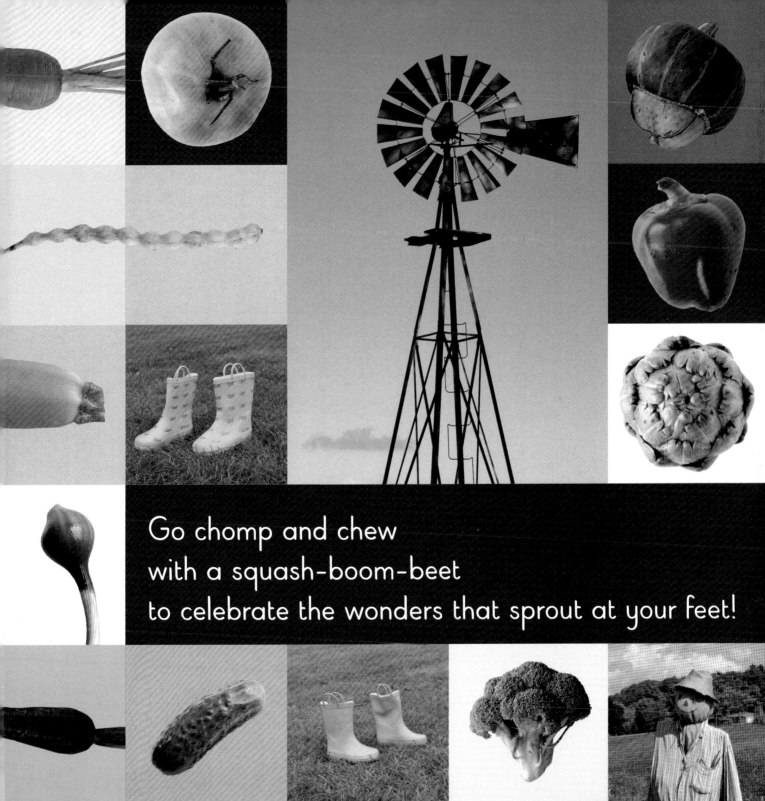

Go chomp and chew
with a squash-boom-beet
to celebrate the wonders that sprout at your feet!

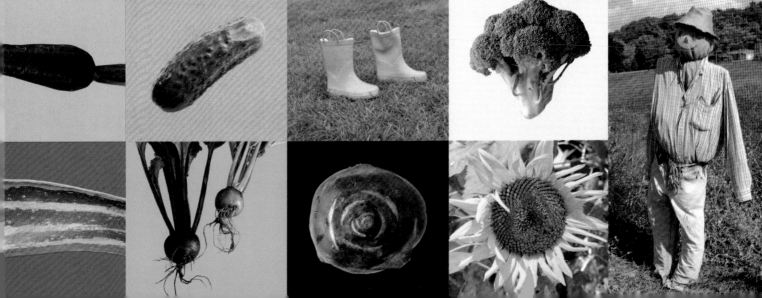

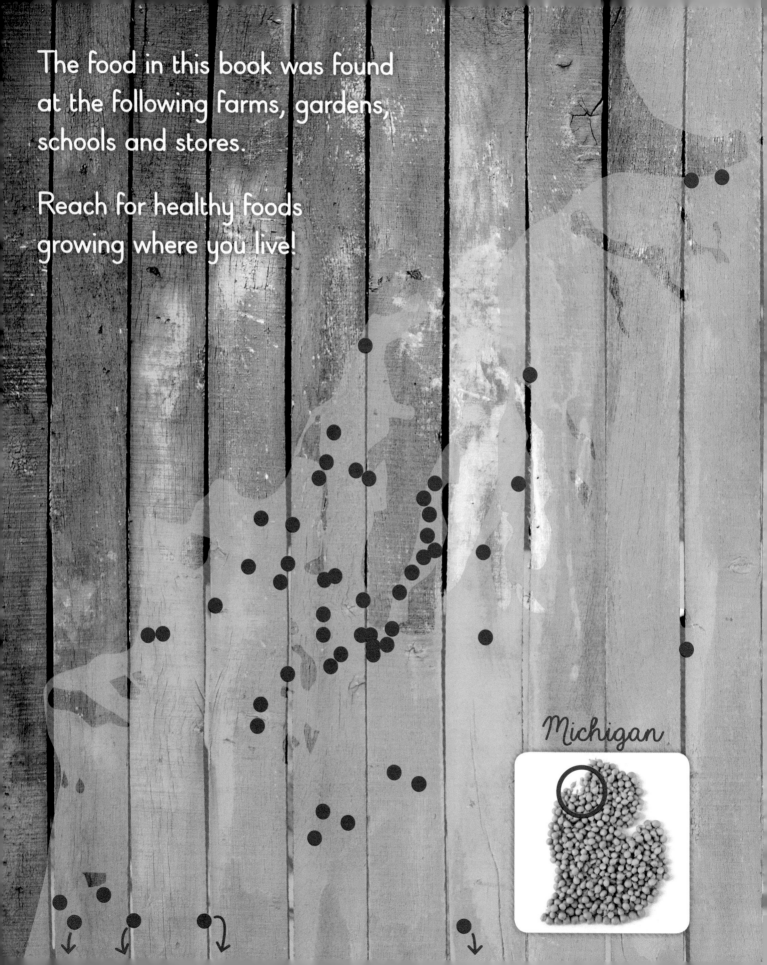

The food in this book was found
at the following farms, gardens,
schools and stores.

Reach for healthy foods
growing where you live!

Michigan

9 Bean Rows

Altonen Orchards

Bardenhagen Farms

Bare Knuckle Farm

Bear Creek Organic Farm

Between the Bays: Warren Orchards

Birch Point Farm

Bootstrap Farms

Cedar Sol Hydro Farm

The Cheese Lady

Cherry Beach Orchards

Cherry Republic

The Children's House, montessori school

Coveyou Scenic Farm Market

Daddy's Girls Fruits and Vegetables

Family Thyme Farm

First Congregational Church & Community
    Children's Center gardens

Five Springs Farm

Food For Thought Farm

Forest Garden Organic Farm

Gallagher's Farm Market and Bakery

Greenrock Farm

Holmestead Farm

Home garden of Dewayne Litwiller,
    executive chef at Grand Traverse Area
    Catholic Schools

Home garden of Tim and Kellie Cutler

Howard Farms

La Casa Verde Produce

Little Red Organics

Loma Farm

Lost Lake Farm

Marvin's Garden Spot

Meadowlark Farm

Nicholas Farms and Vineyard

Norconk Farm

Ocanas Farms

Old Hundredth Farm

Old Mission Peninsula School

Olds Farm

Oryana Natural Foods Market

Pahl's Country Store

Pathfinder School

Petal Pushers Greenhouse

Platte River Gardens

Press On Juice

Providence Organic Farm

Ralph Schaub Farm

Second Spring Farm

Shiloh's Garden

Still Point Farm

Sweeter Song Farm

Tabone Orchards & Vineyards

The Ugly Tomato

Umami Mami

UnderToe Farm

Westmaas Farms

Wunsch Farms

For more information, visit
www.squashboombeet.com.

Farm Field Notes

1.

2.

3.

4.

5.

6.

Add photos, lists or drawings of the fun foods you have discovered!